Anxiety

A Beginner's Guide to Deal with It

© Copyright 2017 by _____ - All rights reserved.

The following book is reproduced below with the goal of providing information that is as accurate and as reliable as possible. Regardless, purchasing this book can be seen as consent to the fact that both the publisher and the author of this book are in no way experts on the topics discussed within, and that any recommendations or suggestions made herein are for entertainment purposes only. Professionals should be consulted as needed before undertaking any of the action endorsed herein.

This declaration is deemed fair and valid by both the American Bar Association and the Committee of Publishers Association and is legally binding throughout the United States.

Furthermore, the transmission, duplication or reproduction of any of the following work, including precise information, will be considered an illegal act, irrespective whether it is done electronically or in print. The legality extends to creating a secondary or tertiary copy of the work or a recorded copy and is only allowed with an express written consent of the Publisher. All additional rights are reserved.

The information in the following pages is broadly considered to be a truthful and accurate account of facts, and as such any inattention, use or misuse of the information in question by the reader will render any resulting actions solely under their purview. There are no scenarios in which the publisher or the original author of this work can be in any fashion deemed liable for any hardship or damages that may befall them after undertaking information described herein.

Additionally, the information found on the following pages is intended for informational purposes only and should thus be considered, universal. As befitting its nature, the information presented is without assurance regarding its continued validity or interim quality. Trademarks that mentioned are done without written consent and can in no way be considered an endorsement from the trademark holder.

Table of Contents

Introduction 1

Chapter 1: Understanding the Beast That Is Called Anxiety 3

Chapter 2: Stress and the Physical Body 9

Chapter 3: Signs That Indicate You Are Suffering from Anxiety . 15

Chapter 4: The Different Types of Anxiety That Can Be Diagnosed 23

Chapter 5: The Many Causes of Anxiety.. 31

Chapter 6: Understanding What Triggers You................................. 37

Chapter 7: Your Responsibility in Your Anxiety 41

Chapter 8: Healthy Ways to Approach Your Anxiety..................... 45

Chapter 9: Eliminating Anxiety for the Long-Term........................ 51

Chapter 10: Common Mistakes to Avoid When Navigating Your Stress 57

Conclusion 61

Introduction

Congratulations on purchasing your personal copy of *Anxiety: A Beginner's Guide to Deal with It*. Thank you for doing so.

The following chapters will provide you with information regarding everything that you need to know about your anxiety. These days, an increasing number of people report living with a heightened level of anxiety. If you are reading this book, there's a chance that you also fall into this category. You are not alone; yet, you probably want to figure out a healthy way to both diagnose and deal with your anxiety promptly. That's what this book can offer you.

This book is going to outline various types of anxiety from which you might be suffering, and will also provide you with information in a way that is straightforward and easily understandable. Instead of feeling like your emotions and psychological feelings cannot possibly be understood, you will feel like you know a bit more about what's going on in your head after you finish reading this book. The internal mind does not have to remain a mystery, yet many people do not know where to begin when it comes to sifting through the mind's processes to find greater peace.

The last chapter of this book is going to discuss some mistakes that should be avoided when you are first learning to cope with your anxiety, if and when it does arise. By becoming aware of the various mistakes that others with anxiety typically make, the hope is that you will be less likely to make these same mistakes yourself.

If you can learn how to deal with your anxiety healthily, it's likely that you will feel less overwhelmed by it. If you can develop a greater sense of control over your mind, then anxiety will become less frightening and therefore much more manageable.

There are plenty of other books on the market that have to do with anxiety. Thank you for choosing this one! Enjoy the rest of what this book, *Anxiety: A Beginner's Guide to Deal with It* has to offer, and remember to write a positive review on Amazon if you find the information in this book useful. Thanks again!

Chapter 1
Understanding the Beast That Is Called Anxiety

Before we begin to look at how you can go about developing techniques that will encourage less anxiety in your life, you first need to understand exactly what anxiety is. That's what this chapter will encompass. After reading this chapter, you will firmly understand what anxiety is. In addition to defining anxiety, this chapter will also seek to understand a brief history of anxiety and how we have come to understand it to the present day. As with any other type of phenomenon, anxiety has a history that has led to how it's perceived in modern day society. By understanding the roots of anxiety, coping with it will become all the more possible, especially when we get into techniques that you can use to combat it.

What is Anxiety?

At its core, anxiety can be defined as a feeling that presents itself as overwhelmingly worrisome. Other words that can be used to describe anxiety include fear, an undefinable tension in the gut, and even excessive nervousness. It's important to understand that in small doses, anxiety is normal. Everyone experiences anxiety due to the pressures of everyday life. This is not uncommon. What is uncommon is when an individual feels anxious on almost a constant basis. Today, it's estimated that over forty-million Americans suffer from some sort of anxiety disorder. We will get into the specific types of anxiety disorders in a subsequent chapter.

Anxiety is Not Always Equal

Another important distinction that needs to be made about anxiety from the onset is that the World Health Organization has determined that not all countries experience anxiety equally. For example, it's estimated that the countries with the highest levels of anxiety include the following:

1. India

2. China

3. The United States

4. Brazil

5. Indonesia

Contrastingly, the countries with the lowest levels of anxiety include the following:

1. Denmark

2. Finland

3. The Netherlands

4. Sweden

5. Ireland

While the highest and lowest levels of anxiety may exist in a particular country for a variety of reasons, it's incredibly interesting to note that higher levels of anxiety can be seen in different parts of the world. This makes anxiety a phenomenon that can change depending on where you live. It also makes anxiety something that can be cured. Understanding this is the first step in curing your own anxiety, as long as you are willing to lessen certain things in your life that cause stress in the first place.

The Discovery of Stress

The ancient Greeks were the first people to discover anxiety, which shouldn't be too much of a surprise considering they are responsible for discovering much of life's most basic principles to this day. When the Greeks first recognized anxiety, however, they did not immediately give it this name. Instead, they described it using the word *hysteric*. Specifically, the ancient Greek term for hysteria was *hysterika*, which can be directly translated to mean *uterus*. This makes sense, as in those days it was determined that only women were affected by the hysteria that anxiety brought with it. Specifically, the ancient Greeks determined that a uterus produced an excess of female semen when a female was not having enough sex in her life. For this reason, it was thought that the only remedy to this ailment was for a woman to engage in more sexual relations as a way to release the hysteria that her semen was producing.

Hysteria through the Years

After the Greeks officially coined a term for stress, other cultures throughout history also came into contact as well. One way that this is apparent is by taking a look at the events of the Salem Witch Trials. These trials took place from the 1500s all the way until the late 1720s. Women, in particular, were seen to be witches when they possessed irrationally high levels of hysteria. A similar phenomenon occurred in the Victorian era in Britain, where women were often taken to insane asylums if they had panic attacks or had other anxiety-related issues. It's not clear whether men can suffer from anxiety until the Civil War when post-traumatic stress disorder was diagnosed amongst soldiers. By the early 1900s, the Russians were the first country to actually treat their soldiers on the battlefield with psychiatrists who went to war with the rest of the military. Finally, we come to the present day, where anxiety is frequently combatted using anxiety medication and antidepressants.

Where Does Anxiety Come From?

If you think about it, anxiety today is far different from anxiety that existed for people living in historical times. For example, not many of us have to worry about hunting our food. If someone goes hunting, they are typically doing it as a sport, not because it's how they survive. Anxiety exists because our ancestors had to deal with stressors related to their livelihood. They could be easily attacked if they weren't on high alert, or if they weren't protecting themselves properly. In this way, it's easy to see how the body used anxiety to bring greater awareness to a person's surroundings. Today, our anxiety is different than what it was when it was first being used by humans. We may have anxiety because we're worried we're going to lose our job, or we have emotional family problems that we have to deal with.

How Does Anxiety Feel?

Even though you might know that you have a lot of anxiety on a regular basis, it still might be difficult to define it in your own terms. On average, people who have some sort of anxiety problem experience these feelings on a regular basis:

1. **Excessive worrying**: This worrying might come from watching the news, or it might turn on whenever your child leaves the house. The worrisome thoughts will not go away, no matter how hard you try to make them disappear.

2. **Muscle Cramps**: Another sign that you might have too much anxiety is if your muscles often feel cramped or tight. This tension can form in the jaw, through clenching your fists or even biting the inside of your cheek. You might think that these are simply bad habits you need to break, but the fact of the matter is that it could be a sign that you suffer from anxiety.

3. **An Unbalanced Gut:** Irritable Bowel Syndrome, also known as IBS, often goes hand-in-hand with anxiety. Even though you may have never thought about it, your gut is actually quite sensitive when you feel anxiety coming on. Other digestive issues other than IBS can also be the result of anxiety. In fact, even a simple upset stomach can be a sign that you are experiencing more anxiety than usual.

The First Signs that Anxiety is Coming

These three can be seen as the most common signs of anxiety, but there are other, less noticeable, signs that can also tell you that you are experiencing it. These first signs include:

1. A shortness of breath

2. A feeling of lightheadedness

3. A headache or migraine

4. Sweating, especially if it's not hot out

5. A pounding in your heart

Again, anxiety is quite common. Everyone experiences the first signs of anxiety from time to time, but you may still want to lessen anxiety in your life whenever you can. We all want to lead stress-free and happy lives, and sometimes our anxiety can make this seem impossible. Understanding the history of anxiety can help to show that anxiety has been around since the beginning of time. Our body naturally produces anxiety as a way to tell our brain that our body may be in danger. There are plenty of ways to reduce anxiety, and it's important to realize that anxiety is something that you can control to some degree. With the right guidance and knowledge, you will soon be able to lessen anxiety in your life in a positive and permanent way.

Chapter 2
Stress and the Physical Body

The previous chapter was hopefully able to define stress for you through a variety of historical lenses; however, these historical facts should not negate the fact that anxiety is an actual occurrence that takes place within an individual's body. This chapter is going to discuss how stress can influence the body, and what the brain is doing during the times when you feel the most stress in your life. After reading this chapter, you will have a basic understanding of the body's processes when you are undergoing high levels of stress. By being able to identify how your body reacts to stress, you should be able to recognize when you are feeling more anxious than usual. If you can understand this, you can then take a step back when you are in a stressful situation and possibly calm yourself down before a panic attack or another sign of anxiety strikes.

The Hypothalamus and the Body's Nervous Systems

Within the body, there exist two types of nervous systems that have to do with stress. Collectively, they are known as the autonomic nervous system. Separately, they are known as the parasympathetic nervous system, and the sympathetic nervous system. While both are certainly important aspects of the human body, the sympathetic nervous system is going to be more important for the purposes of our discussion; however, understanding what the parasympathetic nervous system does is still important. The parasympathetic nervous system is primarily responsible for the regulation of various parts of our bodily functions. Some of these functions include:

1. Regulating digestion
2. Keeping the heart rate down
3. Regulating the intestinal system

In contrast to the functions of the parasympathetic nervous system, the sympathetic nervous system does the opposite. In fact, you have probably heard of the sympathetic nervous system before but may not know it. The sympathetic nervous system is also known as your body's "fight or flight response." In other words, it produces your body's responses when you feel like you are in a stressful or potentially threatening circumstance. These responses directly contrast the functions of the parasympathetic nervous system. When in harmony, these two nervous symptoms balance the body, but when you are feeling tense, this balance becomes completely out of sync. Your fight or flight response is what kicks your anxiety into high-alert. Often, a person like you or me may not even be able to tell that the body is automatically going into fight or flight. For this reason, it's important that you are aware of the signs that will tell you when this occurs. Signs that your fight or flight response has started include the following:

Sign 1 that Your Fight or Flight Response Has Jumpstarted into Action: Developing Tunnel Vision

When this happens, it's almost as if you cannot see out of your peripheral vision. Dizziness or being able to only focus on one thing at a time can accompany a tunnel-vision reaction to something.

Sign 2 that Your Fight or Flight Response Has Jumpstarted into Action: Greater Sensitivity to Noise

Another, subtle, sign that your body has gone into fight or flight is if you notice that you can hear noises that are low in volume or intensity.

Sign 3 that Your Fight or Flight Response Has Jumpstarted into Action: Enlarged Pupils

If you see someone with pupils that are larger than normal, especially when it's perfectly bright outside, this can be one indicator that their body feels particularly stressed at that moment. You can think about the sympathetic nervous system as being connected to our most primal feelings of safety. Before the days when electricity and lighting were easily accessible, the human body needed to adapt to certain situations when there was an immediate threat within their vicinity. One of the ways to do this was to heighten vision through an enlargement of the pupils.

Sign 4 that Your Fight or Flight Response Has Jumpstarted into Action: Pale and Chilly Skin

When your sympathetic nervous system is pumping out cortisol in high doses, this means that it's using energy that would otherwise be used to do things such as heat the body and provide it with a vital glow. Instead of this energy being used to heat the body, it's going to be used to provide more energy to your extremities, eyes, and ears. This way, your body will be on high alert in case it needs to act and move quickly.

Sign 5 that your Fight or Flight Response Has Jumpstarted into Action: A Dry Mouth

Another telltale sign that you are experiencing stress and that your sympathetic nervous system has begun to work overtime is that your mouth is going to feel excessively dry. This is especially true if your body is in the process of digesting something that you recently ate. Similar to when the body saves its energy and causes you to look paler and feel cooler, it's also going to stop digesting food if an immediate stressor becomes apparent. With the stoppage of digestion will come the stoppage of saliva to the mouth, which will result in a dry sensation.

As you can see from the examples of what happens when your body's fight or flight response is triggered, your body is going to change when it's under a lot of anxiety. When these changes are brief, there's not a whole lot of problems that will occur over the long-term. In fact, the body is hard-wired to experience and deal with anxiety every now and then, so it will be able to handle high levels of stress in small doses. On the other hand, problems that can have longer effects on the body can occur if we allow ourselves to undergo large levels of stress over a long period of time. Some of the physical signs that your body is experiencing stress too frequently include the following:

Sign 1 that Your Body's Been Stressed for Too Long: General Fatigue

General fatigue can be best defined as feeling tired during the day even when you have got a good night sleep the night before. You can also experience general fatigue if you feel tired during the evening when you are trying to go to sleep, but cannot seem to fall asleep, no matter how hard you try.

Sign 2 that Your Body's Been Stressed for Too Long: Weight Gain or Loss

Any type of weight gain or weight loss can indicate to you that your body is experiencing stress too often. This is especially true if there are no other reasons why you are gaining or losing weight. For example, sometimes people gain or lose weight because they recently experienced a death in the family or because they are going through a tough breakup. These are normal reasons for a change in weight. If you do not have anything going on in your life that would lead to a change in your weight, then general anxiety may be the cause.

Sign 3 that Your Body's Been Stressed for Too Long: You Are Getting Sick Often

When your fight or flight response has been turned on, it's going to require more energy than normal so that it can heighten your senses. When this happens, it means that it's going to take energy away from other systems in order body to get the energy that it needs. One area of the body that it takes energy away from is your immune system. When your immune system is down, it's much more likely that you will become sick, with a common cold, the flu, or another type of bacteria that can enter the body.

The Effects of Anxiety on Our Reproductive Organs

Again, it's important to understand that everyone is going to experience anxiety in their life at one time or another, but excessive stress is what you should be looking to avoid. In addition to the potential problems that were just discussed above, some problems that can occur particularly in men include erectile dysfunction and sometimes even complete impotence. For women, the most common sign of excessive anxiety via the reproductive organs is a light or sometimes non-existent menstrual cycle. This can sometimes even lead to more worrying for a woman since a lighter period is also an early sign of pregnancy.

As should be obvious after reading this chapter, there are many different types of phenomenon that take place in the body in reaction to high levels of anxiety. It's not uncommon for people to simply not notice when these things are happening inside of them; however, if you have ever felt your body reacting to anxiety in one of the ways that were mentioned above, then you already have an awareness of how uncomfortable this can be. Having a grounded, fully functioning body is one of the key fundamental elements of leading a healthy life; yet as our environments become increasingly filled with stress, functioning within a stressful environment sometimes seems like it's becoming the norm instead of the exception. This is not normal, and you should constantly be working against feeling like it is.

Chapter 3
Signs That Indicate You Are Suffering from Anxiety

While the information in the previous chapter is helpful when you are seeking to understand how anxiety influences the body from a biological perspective, the truth of the matter is that it can be hard to identify the changes that are taking place within the body, especially if you are stressed while they are occurring. For example, it can be a bit difficult to notice that your skin has become paler and chillier to the touch, especially if you haven't had the time to look at yourself in a mirror. This chapter is going to outline some of the more obvious signs that can exist when your anxiety is taking a noticeable toll on you. These signs will include ones that have to do with your mental state, your relationships, and even your ability to complete tasks on a daily basis. The signs that we're going to look at in this chapter will be much more obvious than the biological ones at which we looked in the previous chapter.

The Mental Signs of Anxiety

Before we get into other aspects of your life that anxiety can negatively influence, we will begin this chapter by examining the mind. One of the first ways that you may personally notice heightened levels of anxiety that are affecting you is through your internal monologue with yourself. Some of the mental signs that can indicate that stress is taking a toll on you include the following:

Mental Sign of Anxiety 1: Restlessness

If you have ever laid in bed for what seems like hours on end, with your mind constantly racing, then you have experienced the side-effect of stress that is restlessness. This can often be one of the first indicators that stress is taking a toll on your mind in the form of overactive and constant thoughts. Contrastingly, if you are experiencing the desire to sleep too much, this too can be a sign of excessive anxiety. Remember, when you are stressed, your body is going to be using energy disproportionately. This can certainly cause you to feel more tired than normal. Lastly, restlessness does not necessarily mean that you are either not sleeping or sleeping too much. Restlessness can also manifest itself as causing you to sleep for just a few hours, before waking up or tossing and turning throughout the night.

Mental Sign of Anxiety 2: Irritability

Of course, if you are having trouble sleeping, this can certainly result in feeling increasingly irritable on a day-to-day basis. The biggest way that irritability can negatively affect someone who is experiencing stress is through their relationships. Often, irritable people do not even notice that they are irritable because they are only irritable when they are around others. When they are alone, everything appears to be fine. If you are worried that you might be projecting irritability onto others, you should try to look inward and diagnose your irritability. This way, you can at least attempt to be more pleasant around the people that you care about and interact with often.

Mental Sign of Anxiety 3: Compulsive Behaviors

Even though compulsive behaviors can be considered actions rather than mental thoughts, this type of behavior often comes from a place of mental instability. For example, if you are subconsciously stressing about leaving your house for one reason or another, this may result in you feeling like you *must* clean your house in a meticulous manner prior to doing so. The compulsion to clean your house is a behavioral response to the mental anxiety that you are experiencing, rather than a behavior in its own right.

Mental Sign of Anxiety 4: Forgetfulness

Forgetfulness can be similar to compulsive behavior because forgetting to do something can be just as compulsive as a repetitive behavior. For example, let's say that you are someone who still has anxiety about leaving your house, but instead of cleaning, you forget to bring something along with you after you have already left the house instead. This can result in you feeling like you *must* go back to your house, and then ultimately makes you feel like you have wasted so much time that there's no point in leaving the house again. This means that if you typically categorize yourself as a forgetful person, it might be wise to look inward in an attempt to figure out whether you are truly forgetting, or if some other mental stress is lying just beneath the surface.

Mental Sign of Anxiety 5: Memory Problems

Forgetfulness is different from experiencing memory problems. When you are experiencing memory problems, it's likely that you will have difficulty recalling events that have taken place over the short-term. Often, a traumatic event is also going to trigger memory loss, because the brain is trying to protect itself from experiencing this pain repeatedly. Additionally, it's important to note that what can initially be restlessness can turn into memory issues, because being tired can often result in the brain lacking its memory capabilities.

The Relationship-Related Signs of Anxiety

In additional to personal symptoms of anxiety that can exist in the mind, when you are feeling anxious on a frequent basis, the health of your relationships will also likely be compromised. For some of us, the deterioration of our relationships can sometimes be even more devastating than the mental unclarity that is coming to light. When we see people whom we love pulling away from us, it can be understandably scary and cause even more anxiety to come to the forefront of our brains than already exists. For this reason, it's important to be able to notice when your actions may be indicating that your anxiety is causing your relationships to become potentially jeopardized. The signs that anxiety could be ruining your relationships include the following:

Relationship Anxiety Sign 1: You are "Vegging Out" More than You Are Going Out

One of the first indicators that stress is causing you to back away from your relationships can often be if you suddenly are less excited about spending time with others. For example, if you typically spend most of your weekends out and about with friends, but have noticed that you are spending a lot more time alone lately, then this can be a sign that anxiety is plaguing your normal relationship habits. Sure, if you are going through a breakup or have had some other stressful situation recently occur, then it's perhaps normal for you to feel yourself pulling away from others for at least a little while. On the other hand, if you can recognize that this shift in your behavior is something that is slowly becoming the norm rather than the exception, it might be time to either seek professional help or determine what the root cause of this stress is so that you can rectify the situation in which you find yourself.

Relationship Anxiety Sign 2: An Underactive Libido

We touched on this briefly in the previous chapter, but another surefire sign that anxiety is making your relationships more difficult is if you are experiencing problems in the bedroom. For example, you might be trying to please your partner in the bedroom, but often come away from the sexual experience feeling like you were simply going through the motions the entire time it was occurring. This can be frightening for any relationship, especially because a decline in sexual satisfaction is one of the first signs that a relationship might be in trouble. It's important to understand that just because you do not necessarily feel physically attracted to your partner, this does not mean that your relationship is going to fall apart. Anxiety can often cloud our ability to love our partner adequately, but this does not mean that this feeling of unattraction will last forever.

Relationship Anxiety Sign 3: Moodiness

Another sign that anxiety might be taking more of a toll on you than you initially thought is if you are finding that more than one person has commented on your moodiness. Of course, when someone tells you that you are being moody, you may initially become defensive or want to become argumentative with that person; however, if there's more than one person informing you that they believe you are being moodier than usual, you may want to start being receptive to what they are saying. This is especially true if you are typically not moody. No one wants to be around someone who is constantly changing their emotional demeanor. Additionally, people sometimes will jump to the irrational conclusion that they are developing a bipolar disorder, based on their moodiness. Before you start self-diagnosing yourself with a mental illness, the more appropriate action would be to try and figure out if your moodiness is associated with your anxiety.

Miscellaneous Signs of Anxiety

In addition to the mental and relationship-related anxiety signs that we've already discussed, there are a few other warning signs that can suggest you have got too much anxiety on your plate. These symptoms can manifest themselves in the following ways:

1. **Obsessing Over Irrational Fears:** If you have ever met someone with a phobia, then you know someone who lives with an irrational fear. While irrational fears are often fears that began when an individual was young, excessive worrying is also often associated with older people who have too much time on

their hands. This is similar to become stir crazy after being in your house for too long a period of time. These days, irrational fears can seem even more apparent than ever before, for the simple reason that the news seems to love featuring stories that are sensationalistic in nature.

2. **Experiencing Panic Attacks:** People can experience panic attacks for a variety of reasons, but at their core, they are typically caused by either a need that is not being met in a person's life or the realization of something during a stressful period of time. These types of attacks can often last for minutes and are accompanied by difficulty breathing, stomach cramps, and even an excessive heart rate. It's important to note that just because you have one or two panic attacks, this does not mean that you have a serious issue that needs to be addressed; rather, you may simply be going through a particularly difficult period in your life and need to cope with these issues more directly.

3. **Experiencing Flashbacks:** Lastly, anxiety can often come from experiences from the past that have left a lasting impression on the mind and body of a person. This is especially true if that experience negatively manipulated not just the mind of the person, but also touched the individual's physical body in some manner. We will discuss the various types of anxiety disorders in a subsequent chapter, but flashbacks are often related to serious trauma that has occurred in a person's life.

After reading this chapter, you might be thinking to yourself, "Geez, I experience a lot of these symptoms, I must be extremely anxious!" When you are self-examining your mental tendencies, it can become strangely satisfying to determine that you are guilty of all of them and have an anxiety disorder. Prior to reaching that conclusion, you should try and examine your behavior over a longer period of time. For example, you can try documenting your behavioral tendencies for at between two weeks to a month. This will allow you to determine whether or not the behavior you are experiencing is consistent, or it's just something that will pass soon.

Chapter 4
The Different Types of Anxiety That Can Be Diagnosed

Now that you are aware of both the biological and mental tendencies that can occur when you find yourself under a considerable amount of stress, it's time to formally diagnose some of these anxiety-related problems. That's what this chapter will cover. After reading this chapter, you will have a better understanding of the types of anxiety disorders with which people are commonly diagnosed. It's important to note here that while this chapter will discuss various types of anxiety disorders at length, these descriptions should not be used as a replacement for a formal diagnosis from a doctor. Self-diagnosing yourself is always going to be a slippery slope, especially if you turn out to be wrong about what you are experiencing.

Not All Anxiety is the Same

Before we begin to look at the various types of anxieties with which a person can be diagnosed, it's important to understand that it's entirely possible for a person to possess tendencies that exist within multiple disorder categories. As a society, the easiest way to explain and understand a disorder is through generalizations; however, these generalizations should not always be taken literally. For each of the types of anxieties that we're going to discuss, keep in mind that there is always going to be a spectrum of it that a person will fall into. Along these same lines, it's also possible for an individual to suffer from multiple anxiety disorders at the same time. If you are reading this book because you want to know more about the anxiety that you are experiencing, be patient with yourself. Even if you have multiple types of anxiety disorders, it's going to be okay as long as you actively seek out the help that you need.

Information Regarding Generalized Anxiety Disorder

Commonly referred to as GAD, generalized anxiety disorder is the most commonly diagnosed anxiety disorder that exists today. In fact, there are millions of people that deal with GAD throughout the world, let alone in the United States. The phrase "generalized" in the name of the disorder itself is intentional and refers to the fact that this type of anxiety never quite goes away. Instead, it buzzes in the back of a person's mind, always on autopilot and never taking a break. This type of anxiety can present itself in the form of constant worrying, constant stress, and an incessant tension. Yes, dealing with anxiety is an aspect of life with which everyone has to cope, but when this anxiety seems to be for no apparent reason, GAD may be the cause. Some of the primary symptoms that a person with GAD will experience include the following:

1. **Overthinking:** A person with GAD will often experience what are known as "catastrophic" thoughts. These are thoughts that focus on the negative and will not go away, no matter what.

2. **Low Levels of Energy:** A person with GAD will also experience lethargy on a semi-constant basis for seemingly no

reason. This does not count if you are someone who enjoys going on long distant runs on frequently. It only accounts for people who are tired even though they have not done much of anything.

3. **An Inability to Focus:** This symptom pretty much speaks for itself, and includes forgetting what you are saying in mid-conversation and not being able to stay on task for a long period of time.

4. **Muscle Tension:** A person with GAD is often going to experience muscle tension, particularly in the upper half of the body including the neck, the back, and the shoulder blades.

Remember, a key to being diagnosed with GAD is that these symptoms are occurring without much pause on a regular basis. In addition to GAD being the most popularly diagnosed form of anxiety, it's also the disorder that is most often diagnosed with other anxiety disorders simultaneously. Typically, the two other types of disorders that GAD is commonly associated with are panic and compulsive-related ones.

Obsessive Compulsive Disorder

Speaking of compulsion, the next type of anxiety-related disorder we're going to discuss is the Obsessive-Compulsive Disorder or OCD. While OCD can exist on a scale and may not be incredibly damaging to the person who is suffering from it, the possibility also exists for OCD to confuse and bring fear to an individual's mental facilities. OCD is two-fold in the sense that both the obsessive qualities and the compulsive qualities of the disorder are unique in their own right. The obsessive portion of the disorder primarily has to do with a person's thoughts. The same thought will occur repeatedly in the person's head, and it is often not a thought that is positive in nature. Instead, these thoughts are typically rooted in fear.

Post-Traumatic Stress Disorder

Post-traumatic stress disorder, also known as PTSD, is often associated with people who have served in the military; however, this disorder can also affect people who have never been in combat. For both people who have served in the military and those who have not, PTSD is characterized by stress that occurs because of a traumatic event that took place in the past. This event can be either emotional or physical in nature, but more often than not it is a physical event to which a person had an extremely emotional response. It's also important to note that in some cases, people who have witnessed a traumatic event can also be diagnosed with this anxiety disorder. For example, witnessing a death or watching a friend suffer in some manner. Some signs of PTSD in an individual include the following:

1. **Emotional Instability:** Specifically, people with PTSD often deal with feelings involving isolation, numbness, and detachment from the people who love them. Along these same lines, a person with PTSD may feel like their future is pointless or without purpose.

2. **Stimulus Issues:** Another telling sign that someone has PTSD is if the person responds poorly to a certain stimulus in his or her environment. For example, if the individual who is suffering from PTSD was in the military, their stress related to the event might get triggered from certain loud noises or bright lights. These types of stimuli are known as triggers, and they typically are associated with the event that was traumatic to the person in the first place.

A Fear of the Public, or Agoraphobia

Agoraphobia is a type of anxiety that an individual experiences when he or she is afraid to go out in public. Yes, this anxiety can technically fall under that of any other phobia; however, is often more detrimental to a person's daily life than are other types of phobias that exist. This makes sense when you think about the fact that it's much easier for a person to avoid spiders than it is for a person to completely avoid people on the street or in their workplace. As we've already stated, many types of anxiety disorders can combine with others. Many people with agoraphobia also tend to experience anxiety related to PTSD or panic disorders. We will be discussing panic disorders next. Agoraphobia is more common in adults than it is for younger people. Some other symptoms related to agoraphobia include the following:

1. **Stress when Socializing:** When in social settings, a person suffering from agoraphobia will likely feel incredibly anxious and uncomfortable; however, the other people around this person may not be aware of this sense of discomfort.

2. **Control-Related Anxiety:** Another symptom of agoraphobia has to do with control. Often, people with agoraphobia enjoy controlling their environment. When they are unable to control every single stimulus that's occurring, stress can ensue.

3. **Safety Concerns:** When an agoraphobic does find him or herself out in public, they are likely thinking about ways that they can find shelter in case something terrible happens. In other words, these types of safety concerns will be accompanied by thoughts of impending doom.

Panic Anxiety Disorder

Similar to agoraphobia and PTSD, a panic anxiety disorder can be extremely incapacitating to a person, especially because of the physical symptoms that accompany this disorder. When someone has a panic disorder, it's often triggered by stressful mental thoughts; however, it's also possible for a person who is suffering from a panic disorder to simply feel panic because they are worried about potentially having another panic attack. A panic attack can be described as a powerful bodily response that shakes a person to their core. When a person has a panic attack, the following will often occur:

1. Difficulty breathing

2. Pain in the chest or abdomen

3. Heaving and sobbing

4. A feeling of lightheadedness, or even an "out of body" sensation

5. An increased heart rate

While reading these symptoms, you might be thinking to yourself, "wow, people who have panic disorders are a tad dramatic"; however, for the person experiencing a panic attack these symptoms are incredibly real and jarring. In addition to these very real physical sensations, mental problems often always accompany the physical symptoms that an attack will bring. The types of mental thoughts that can occur while a panic attack is ensuing can include thoughts of death and a feeling of complete isolation and helplessness.

Social Anxiety Disorder

Agoraphobia and social anxiety can seem like they have similar symptoms; however, social anxiety differs from agoraphobia in the sense that social anxiety often affects a person even when they are socializing with their friends in smaller circles. Additionally, an individual will experience more paranoia when they are dealing with social anxiety than they will when they are battling agoraphobia. For example, some clear signs of social anxiety disorder include the following:

1. An intense and often irrational fear of being judged or even stared at by other people in a social setting

2. An extreme fear of speaking in public. Most people have at least some fear when it comes to public speaking, but a person with a social anxiety disorder is going to have excessive fear in these types of situations.

3. An inability to find their voice in social settings. A person who is experiencing social anxiety may even be unable to answer questions when in social circles.

As you can see after reading this chapter, there are many ways that anxiety can be diagnosed, understood, and coped with. Even if you do not think you fall into any of these distinct stress categories, understanding how people with these disorders operate and think can provide you with a better awareness of how stress manifests in general. When avoided and ignored, it's clear that anxiety can have severe consequences on our relationships, our minds, and even our physical bodies. For this reason, it should be obvious that keeping a healthy mind that is as anxiety-free as possible is one of the most important things that you can do for yourself.

Chapter 5
The Many Causes of Anxiety

While the previous chapter documented how the most common types of anxiety are formally diagnosed, you may still be wondering how individuals get to a place where their anxiety is so apparent in the first place. That will be the topic of this chapter. It's simply misguided to say that people who suffer from high levels of anxiety are living their lives incorrectly. As you will see, there are a variety of factors at work that can lead a person to feel as if their anxiety is something that's too difficult to endure.

Environmental Factors

In many cases, your environment is going to determine the degree to which your anxiety affects you, regardless of the severity of your anxiety within your brain. In other words, if you grow up in an environment where experiencing anxiety is not a common occurrence, then it's unlikely that you will develop anxiety-motivated tendencies. Additionally, your environment alone can cause you to develop an anxiety-related disorder, even if you are not genetically pre-dispositioned to develop one. In fact, there are plenty of studies out there that suggest that it's entirely possible to cure anxiety disorders without the use of medicine at all. It's been proven that it's possible to rectify some of the effects of stress through environmental and behavioral changes alone.

It's obvious that a stressful home environment is going to likely cause a person environmental stress, but it's less obvious that environmental stress can also come from changes in your environment as well. A huge example of an environmental stressor that over fifty-percent of the US population has experienced is the stress that comes with going through a divorce. When you divorce someone, you are forced to completely change and alter the way of life that you are used to living. With divorce also comes concerns about money, children, and even where both parties will live. This is a great example of how changes in your environment can lead to great levels of stress. At the core of this type of stress often lies the desire to feel safe, secure, and loved by the people around you and the ones whom you call your family. Feeling safe is a biological need that all humans have, and this is where much of environmental anxiety begins to take form.

The Emotional Causes of Anxiety

In addition to our physical surroundings causing stress, another way that anxiety can manifest is through our emotions. Emotions have to do with our interactions with other people, how we were raised and how we feel we should be loved. A major way that our emotions can cause anxiety, especially later in life, is if we experienced neglect or abuse when we were younger. Abuse and neglect can fall under the umbrella of both traumatic life experiences as well as environmental anxiety factors, but these types of ongoing situations can cause an individual to feel and experience anxiety disorders far into the future. At the root of most neglectful and abusive experiences, the victim is left feeling emotionally helpless and damaged. Anxiety, along with a host of other emotional responses, will result from this type of environmental condition. When people who experience neglect and abuse develop anxiety from these experiences, anxiety can become a sort of byproduct of the type of response that this individual will have regarding other situations that life throws at them.

In addition to neglect and abuse, traumatic experiences of all types can leave a person feeling emotionally helpless and anxious. Some of the signs of emotional anxiety include the following:

Sign 1 of Emotional Anxiety: Feeling Like Your Mind's a Blank Slate

The inability to think at all is one sign of emotional anxiety. If you have ever experienced a situation where you cannot seem to recall anything when you need to, this is an example of emotional anxiety at work. By thinking about nothing, your brain is trying to shield itself from the pain that it's likely experienced in the past due to an emotionally-trying experience. Not being able to concentrate is another way that emotional anxiety presents itself in people.

Sign 2 of Emotional Anxiety: Expecting the Worst

A general feeling of pessimism is another sign that you have experienced some type of emotional trauma in the past. It may be that you are always expecting the worst to happen because your brain is preparing itself in case the worst occurs. In addition to always being on the lookout for the worst to happen, you may also approach situations with dread or extreme apprehension in your head.

Sign 3 of Emotional Anxiety: Irritability

If you do not consider yourself an irritable person, yet often find yourself becoming irritated with situations or with the people around you, then you have experienced irritability stemming from emotional anxiety. Irritability often comes from a place where a person feels uncomfortable because he or she cannot control a situation. Control is a key reason why people often experience emotional anxiety, because they are afraid of being hurt, abused, or emotionally neglected like they were in the past.

Social Anxiety

The last primary cause of anxiety that we're going to look at is social anxiety. Social anxiety can be best defined as a fear that presents itself when you are in social situations. Some key signs of a social anxiety disorder include the following symptoms:

1. **Trouble Talking to Others:** People with social anxiety disorders often will not be able to talk to new people. They might freeze up, or seem incredibly awkward when presented with the opportunity to make new friends.

2. **Trouble Going to New Social Events:** Another key sign of a social anxiety disorder is when a person psyches themselves out of attending a social gathering with a group of people they have never met before or know little about. Rather than looking at this situation as an opportunity to meet new people

and grow their social circle, someone with social anxiety will feel nothing but dread about the social situation. Many times, this will result in the person avoiding the social gathering at all costs.

The two signs above are the most common signs of a social anxiety disorder. Physical body signs that a person suffers from social anxiety include the following:

1. Trouble speaking to the point that no words come out
2. A trembling or shaking in the limbs while in social circles
3. Blushing, even when there is nothing to be embarrassed about

Similar to emotional anxiety that can alter the way in which a person interacts with someone else, social anxiety typically comes from a situation where the person experienced social trauma in the past. For this reason, their brain and body are on high alert and often eager to distance themselves from social situations because of the humiliation or problems that social settings have presented in the past.

Your Lifestyle Can Cause Anxiety

Lastly, your lifestyle can play a larger role than you may think when it comes to how much anxiety you experience daily. One of the most prevalent ways that anxiety can differ between people with different lifestyles revolves around how often they exercise. People who exercise more frequently are far less likely to experience high levels of stress. On the other hand, people who rarely work out will often have a more difficult time dealing with their anxiety. When you think about our bodies as being able to store energy, it's easy to see how unused energy can cause an individual to overthink or build up in an unhealthy manner. When your mind is tired, it has less time to worry.

In addition to living an active lifestyle, eating unhealthily and drug and alcohol use can cause a person to feel more angst and stress. Caffeine also plays a role in heightening feelings related to anxiety. It's important to note that while eating unhealthy food on its own may not directly lead to stress, the feelings that often accompany unhealthy eating can certainly make a person feel anxious. For example, many people feel stress regarding their physical figure or feelings of lethargy after finishing an unhealthy meal. In extreme situations, anxiety related to a person's lifestyle can even cause this person to become anorexic or engage in illicit drug use on a frequent basis.

Chapter 6
Understanding What Triggers You

Having a general understanding of the different types of anxiety that exists and why this anxiety occurs is great; however, if you are unable to identify specific triggers that cause your unique anxiety in your life, then I think we can agree that it is going to be rather difficult to develop anxiety-alleviation techniques for yourself. This chapter is going to document, in a step-by-step fashion, how you can go about identifying what triggers your anxiety in your everyday life.

Step 1 to Understanding Your Anxiety: Identify Your Comfort Zone

When you are first trying to figure out what is making you so anxious, you should think about circumstances in your life where you feel out of place or less than yourself. To do this, you can compare how you feel when you are alone to how you feel around certain people in your life. For example, if you have a significant other, evaluate how they make you feel in relation to how you feel when you are alone. When you are with members of your family or with friends, you can also use this technique. You can use this same barometer to gauge how you feel in different locations daily. For example, is it your living space that's stressing you out, or maybe the type of work that you are doing? By asking yourself these questions, you may be surprised to find easy answers.

Additionally, you can also identify your own discomfort through the analysis of your physical body. This may be harder to identify when you are trying to use self-examination techniques, but some physical body language signs of discomfort include the following:

1. Rubbing of the neck, face, or legs

2. Physically pulling away from someone or blocking them with your arms

3. Crossing your arms or legs

4. The positioning of your feet. If your feet are pointed towards someone during a conversation, you are comfortable. If they are pointed away, you are probably not feeling fully content

5. Eye contact. If you notice that you have trouble looking someone in the eye during a conversation, this may be a sign that you are uncomfortable, even if you are consciously not feeling uneasy

Step 2 to Understanding Your Anxiety: Exercise

One of the best ways to gauge how severe your anxiety truly is can be done through an increase in physical activity. If you are already an active person daily, then you can skip this step, but if you are someone who generally avoids most physical activity, then figuring out how you can exercise in a way that's personally fulfilling can be a great indicator of how well your anxiety responds to exercise. It's important to keep in mind that if you decide to exercise in a way that is not personally fulfilling to you, the physical activity itself can end up causing additional, rather than less, anxiety.

Step 3 to Understanding Your Anxiety: Check Your Diet

Similar to exercising on a more frequent basis, another way to figure out if your lifestyle is contributing to higher-than-normal levels of anxiety is to analyze your diet. Does your diet consist of mostly whole proteins and vegetables, or are you guilty of binging on junk food whenever you can? It's been proven that people who eat healthy diets possess lower levels of depression, anxiety, and other types of problems. For this reason, it's advised that you do not discount the effects that your diet can have on your mental health.

Step 4 to Understanding Your Anxiety: Track Your Sleep

Not getting enough sleep can cause a lot more problems, in addition to anxiety. Some of these problems include weight gain, irritability, acne, and much more. When you are initiating this step, you should try to get a good night's sleep for an entire week. To do this, exercising, limiting your caffeine and sugar intake, and eating healthier foods are all habits that can help to achieve better sleep. If after a week of peacefully sleeping, you have noticed your anxiety has diminished, then you will know that a lack of sleep has been contributing to your problem all along.

Step 5 to Understanding Your Anxiety: Question Your Social Support Networks

Have you ever encountered "friends" that seem to do nothing except bring you down? While it may be difficult spending an increasing amount of time alone, the reality is that negative social influences on your life can often lead to a lot of anxiety and unrest. Studies have shown that the more social support a person has, the less anxiety they experience on a day-to-day basis. Work hard to surround yourself with people who are supportive, rather than detrimental, to your mental health. Have you ever heard the saying, "you become the company you keep"? This saying exists for a simple reason. It's true.

Of course, if you do ultimately discover that your friends are not providing you with the support that you need, the best advice is to talk to them about it before completely shutting them out of your life. Perhaps your relationship needs a reorientation, rather than a definitive ending. Toxic friends are not worth having, even if they are the only friends that you have got. Learning how to take pride in your relationships and find value in them starts with recognizing that you yourself are worth being surrounded by positive, rather than negative, people.

Chapter 7
Your Responsibility in Your Anxiety

By better understanding your tendencies, you should be able to bring greater awareness to your strengths and weaknesses in relation to why your anxiety manifests itself. This next chapter is going to shift attention away from your behavioral tendencies and will instead focus on your mental tendencies. Often, a component of stress and anxiety has to do with guilt surrounding how we as individuals cope with it. For example, if you have ever lashed out at someone angrily, only to realize that it was your anxiety that was motivating you to act in this manner, then you already have some insight on how feelings of guilt can come from feelings of uncertainty, fear, trauma, and pain.

Anxiety Revealing Itself as Anger

It's important to first understand that anger is *always* a secondary emotion. To put it another way, when you become angry it is always going to be because of a feeling of fear, isolation, sadness or pain. Anger itself is not a primary emotion. It's merely a conduit for another emotion that is looking for a little love and attention. Sometimes, anger can be surprising or unanticipated, especially when there is anxiety underneath the surface that's motivating this anger to present itself. This makes anger something that cannot always be easily controlled. For this reason, guilt can often accompany the aftermath of an angry outburst, especially if the person at whom you are directing your anger did not deserve your outburst in the first place.

We can all agree that guilt is a terrible emotion to feel. If you can think back to a situation where you used anger as a way to voice feelings of anxiety, then you can see how overtime guilt can become associated with your anxiety to some degree. When this happens, it's likely that someone who is experiencing stress may begin to think that their feelings of anxiety are entirely their fault; however, all they should really feel guilty for is the way in which they have handled their anxiety in the form of anger, rather than for the anxiety itself. This can certainly confuse the mind, and more importantly can also cause you to feel even more anxious than you previously did.

Walk Away

In addition to reorienting the way that you process guilt in relation to anger and anxiety, another great tactic to use when you are beginning to feel like an angry outburst is coming is to simply walk away from the situation. It might seem cliché to give the advice of, "go blow off some steam," but sometimes walking away from a situation for a brief period of time can provide you and the situation in which you find yourself with a lot more clarity and calm. Over time, it's likely that you will be able to better control your anger to the point where you will not even need to walk away from a situation to feel less angry. Instead, you will be able to cope with your feelings of anger in real-time, which will also provide you with a greater sense of confidence, and less anxiety.

In thinking about these types of emotions and your capacity to understand them, it can be easy to conclude that you are fully to blame for your feelings of anxiety. We've already gone over the different factors that can lead a person to develop an anxiety disorder, so you logically know that anxiety is often not entirely the fault of the person who is experiencing it; however, at the end of the day, you are still responsible for handling your anxiety in the best way that you can. It's pretty obvious that becoming irrationally angry and feeling unwarranted guilt is only going to enhance, rather than help, your anxiety-related problems.

Taking Responsibility Properly

With an awareness of the fact that you are not to blame for the anxiety that you feel, it's still important that you deal with your anxiety properly. We will tackle anger first. The best way to think about anger in relation to your anxiety is to fully accept that you are in complete control of it. Becoming outwardly angry is a choice. Instead of becoming angry without thinking, a better way to deal with it is to consider why you are becoming heated before exploding. Think about the secondary emotion that is prompting the anger. Try to focus on a response that communicates the primary feeling, instead of the angry one.

Anxiety as it Relates to Depression

In addition to feelings of anger, anxiety can often cause a depressive response in individuals as well. In fact, many people report experiencing depression due to anxiety quite frequently. These types of responses include ones that express, "Poor me", "I do not have any friends", or "I'll never amount to anything." Even though these types of thoughts can seem overwhelming, you can also overcome them as a way to better cope with the anxiety that you are feeling.

The best way to deal with these types of depressive thoughts is to take responsibility for them. At the end of the day, no one in this world owes you anything. You are the only person who is responsible for your wellbeing. When you place your sadness onto other people, it will only make your anxiety worse, because you are likely going to allow yourself to feel let down by people who should not have to worry about your happiness. If you are prone to thinking this way, some thoughts and mantras that you can use to cope with these intrusive thoughts include "What do I bring to this situation?", "How can I enhance my experience with this person?" and "I am responsible for my own happiness."

The point of this chapter was to help you to recognize that your anxiety is not your fault. Nonetheless, you still need to hold yourself accountable for the actions that you take due to the anxiety that has been quite unfairly thrust upon you. Anger, guilt, and depression are three of the major ways that anxiety can cause a person to feel and behave. Hopefully, this chapter has been able to help you to recognize some tips that you can use to better navigate anxiety when it wants to come roaring out of you in those three negative emotional forms.

Chapter 8
Healthy Ways to Approach Your Anxiety

You have probably heard the saying, "attitude is everything" at some point in your life. Sure, there's a chance that this saying may have made you roll your eyes once or twice (I'm pretty sure it's made mine do that), but there is value to take from this cliché, especially when it comes to dealing with anxiety. This chapter is going to focus on the types of attributes you should be seeking to develop as someone who is actively working towards diminishing anxiety from their life.

Set Your Intention

As with any new pursuit, acknowledging the goal that you'd like to reach is often the first step towards achieving it. Overcoming anxiety is no different. When you are setting your intention to overcome it, it's important that you also take some time to reflect on how much you dislike the anxiety that you feel and why. By recognizing what you do not like about your current situation, it will relay to you the importance of why you need to deal with your stress head-on. Feel the anxiety and the discomfort that it yields. Recognize its presence.

Love Your Enemy

In addition to recognizing the presence of your anxiety, you should also get comfortable with it. It's typical for people who suffer from excessive anxiety to try and avoid at all costs because anxiety can be a painful sensation to experience. Rather than avoiding it, try to see if you can become comfortable looking your anxiety in the face. Once you can accomplish this, the next step is to look at your anxiety through a nonjudgmental lens. Accomplishing this alone can often alleviate some feelings of anxiety because our own criticisms of ourselves can contribute to our general sense of unease.

Develop an Awareness and Curiosity

In seeking to understand the nuances that exist within your particular anxiety, it's important to pay attention to what's triggering your anxiety to occur in the first place. This is incredibly important. If you do not know exactly why you begin feeling anxious, then you are never going to be able to eliminate this problem from your life and become healthy. When you begin to take notice of what's the root cause of your anxiety, you should do your best to do so in a non-judgmental way. Along these same lines, do not be afraid to ask yourself questions. Analyzing why you behave the way that you do, or why you interact with certain people in your life that way that you do will allow you to truly understand your motives and your thought patterns.

Develop Your Confidence

Overcoming your anxiety is not going to be an easy feat. You will be doing a lot of internal work on yourself, and this is going to require confidence that you may or may not currently possess. A key aspect of developing confidence is learning how to trust yourself. Anxiety can often bring with it feelings of inferiority, hopelessness, and dread. Along these same lines, if your anxiety is coming from a place of trauma, abuse or neglect, guilt from these events can also bring feelings of worthlessness and self-blame. Removing anxiety from your life will require repairing these avenues of misguided and untrue feelings so that fresher and more optimistic feelings can bloom.

Compassion Towards Yourself

Compassion for yourself and your journey goes hand-in-hand with developing your confidence. So often, we have more compassion for other people than we do for ourselves. A great way to practice being more compassionate towards yourself is to try and think about five things that you like about yourself on a daily or semi-weekly basis. If you are currently uncomfortable with complimenting yourself, you can instead begin this practice by simply listing in your head five things that you are thankful for on a daily or semi-weekly basis. This simple activity can bring more optimism into the mind. Being kind to yourself can often yield greater results than you may initially think.

Practice Patience

If you have anxiety since you were a child or grew up in an environment where stress was a major portion of your experience, then there's a chance that you have been practicing the art of being anxious for the majority of your life. Anxiety can be habitual, and it's important that your patient with yourself during the process of dealing with your anxiety more appropriately. Bad habits are hard to break, including emotional ones. For example, if you end up becoming irrationally angry, even though you are trying to work through your emotions more healthily, it's okay. Recognize how you could have handled the situation better and move on. Dwelling on the past will get you nowhere except into the same perpetual cycle of anxiety in which you currently find yourself.

Allow Yourself to Start with a Clean Slate

If you can think about approaching your anxiety from a place of rationalization and are willing to open your eyes to a perspective that you perhaps have not considered in the past, your mind is going to be much more receptive, rather than resistant, to the changes that you are looking to make. An upheaval of your old tendencies is going to require a shift in how you see the world. Take this as an opportunity to grow, and do your best to forego the desire to latch onto old and outdated habits that no longer suit you.

Consider Meditation

You may not think that meditation is for everyone, but to that, I will say that you are wrong. It's been proven that meditation can decrease the effects that anxiety has on the mind, and also possesses a host of other great benefits. You can meditate for as little as two minutes at a time. When you do, focus on your breath. Notice the inhales and the exhales, and do your best to dissuade any other thoughts from coming into your head. Another fabulous way to use meditation, specifically with the goal of decreasing anxiety in mind, is to allow yourself to feel any and all emotions that may come your way during the meditative process. If you can begin to think about your body as a channel that merely processes your emotions, rather than something that internalizes them, it's going to be much easier to let go of past behavioral tendencies that you may have developed in response to anxiety.

Keep Your Body Healthy

We have already briefly discussed how drugs and alcohol could hinder the body's ability to overcome anxiety. In fact, alcohol and drug use can cloud our ability to rid the body of its stress in the first place. When you commit yourself to ridding yourself of your anxiety, you must also dedicate yourself to a lifestyle that is working with, rather than against, good health. For example, yoga is a great way to de-stress and bring greater awareness to your physical body, because when you are doing yoga, you are forced to think about what your body is thinking about and doing. Drinking less caffeine can also help to rid the body of stress. Whatever your vices may be, you should seek to eliminate them as much as you possibly can.

Declutter Your Space

If you live in mess most of the time, it's time that you change this bad habit. Mess can be stressful, it's as simple as that. Studies have shown that people who live amongst constant clutter have a more difficult time concentrating and completing daily tasks than do people who live in a mostly-clean space. Practicing minimalism and other techniques that suggest you get rid of your stuff instead of hoarding it can provide your mind and body with the space that it needs to thrive.

Seek Peace

In addition to decluttering your space, it might also be a good idea to try and bring a greater sense of calm to your home through the inclusion of light and mellowness. For example, you could try to bring more natural light into your home, or you could purchase pictures and home decorations that look soothing to the eye. A great smell that aids in greater calm is lavender. You could try to smell lavender more often. When thinking about how to incorporate more peace into your surroundings, it's the details that matter. What makes you feel at ease? Think about this, and then integrate these details into your home accordingly.

All the tactics that were presented in this chapter can help you to feel more grounded and prepared for eliminating large swaths of anxiety from your life. If you approach your anxiety through these types of techniques, then it's even likely that you will be able to reduce your anxiety prior to even formally doing so. Commit yourself to developing a new and optimistic foundation for which your confidence can grow. From here, wait to see how you feel and what you end up accomplishing within yourself. For journeys that take place within yourself, the changes are often subtle, yet extremely rewarding nonetheless.

Chapter 9
Eliminating Anxiety for the Long-Term

If you feel as if your anxiety is severe, then you may be under the impression that there is nothing that can be done for you except the use of medication. This book is not suggesting that there are no circumstances when a person should seek out the use of medication; however, that type of help is beyond the scope of this book. This chapter is going to focus on remedies that you can use in replacement of medication. After all, if you can solve your anxiety problems without the use of medication, why wouldn't you want to do so?

Talk to Someone

Some people believe that every single person on earth should see a professional psychologist. If you are someone who does not often focus on themselves, paying someone to listen and provide you with advice may be the only opportunity that you have to truly provide yourself with some attention. Do not be afraid to shop around for a psychologist to find someone with whom you mesh well. It's often uncomfortable at times, but if the counselor is good at his or her job, you will soon start to notice changes in yourself after your counseling sessions.

Get Rid of Your Crutches

We've all got vices. Some of us have worse vices than others, but the types of tools that we use as crutches can include drugs, alcohol, sex and even being surrounded by people. If you often feel uncomfortable being alone, then start there. Chisel out some time in your week where you are completely alone. See what happens. If you often use marijuana, more detrimental drugs, or alcohol as a way to distance yourself from your emotions, try to lessen the degree to which you do this. Sex and the use of pornography can also be used as a coping mechanism when performed excessively. Try to evaluate your vices as transparently as possible, and rid yourself of them as necessary. This will allow you to make space for a more positive and emotionally-conscious lifestyle.

Understand that Emotions Are Fleeting

People who can eliminate a lot of anxiety from their lives often successfully do so once they can come to terms with the fact that emotions are fleeting and temporary. This can be a hard thing to recognize, especially when it can seem like our emotions are all-encompassing and strong. Along these same lines, the guilt, feelings of humiliation, and feelings of low self-esteem that you might be feeling at this very moment are ones that are temporary. These are not facts, but rather feelings that are inaccurate. Being able to recognize that these feelings can go away will allow you to feel more motivated and positive when it comes to long-term anxiety relief.

Purposefully Force Your Thoughts Related to Fear

Another, potentially more drastic tactic to use when you are looking to lessen your stress is to force yourself to dwell on whatever scares you and brings anxiety into your head. If you want to try this technique, you will have to be fully committed to it. Otherwise, you will be doing nothing more than focusing on your fears fruitlessly. Set aside a certain amount of time each day to focus on your fears. Think about all aspects of this fear for that allotted period of time. Do this daily. What you will likely find is that over time, this fear is going to lessen in intensity because you have been focusing on it so much. By providing yourself with allotted time to go over your fear in your mind, the goal is that logic will replace any fear that you may be experiencing.

Activity Contest Your Negativity

It's no surprise to anyone who suffers from anxiety that anxiety often brings with it negative thoughts. When these negative thoughts are given attention, they can often be debilitating and stunt any potential for anxiety elimination. A great way to combat a negative thought is to write down the negative thought as soon as you think it. From here, make a list of all the scenarios that are much more likely than the negative one that you have written down. Next, make another list that documents why even if the negative thing happens, it still will not matter. Challenge this thought, until the potential for it to become a reality has been wiped away from your brain. If you have never tried this technique before, it can truly be useful when your worst thoughts have somehow crept to the forefront of your brain without warning.

Create Exciting Memories

Working on your anxiety can sometimes be as stressful as the anxiety that you currently have. For this reason, it's incredibly important that you make sure that you are doing fun things frequently while you work through your stress triggers. This will allow you to create positive memories during this time period, and will also distract you from becoming overwhelmed or anxious about the changes that you desire to make for yourself. When you choose these activities and excursions, you should also seek to do new things whenever you can. Do not be afraid to step outside of your comfort zone. Talk to new people, engage in experiences you have meant to try. Developing new habits as frequently as you can, will make approaching your anxiety all the easier.

Engage in the Art of Self-Care

Self-care relates directly to your confidence. If you have ever walked outside and felt like you are underdressed compared to the men and women on the streets who have their hair done, their clothing pressed, and their shoes shined, then you already know what it feels like to feel less than adequate from a physical perspective. Sometimes, a little bit of self-care can go a long way in easing your anxiety. For example, why not treat yourself to a manicure or a pedicure every now and again? Why not splurge on a massage every three months? When you get these types of treatments done, the message that your brain is receiving is, "I'm good enough. I deserve to be pampered." You want to start trying to cultivate these positive feelings about yourself whenever possible. One day, perhaps you will only have these positive thoughts to think.

Recognize Money Matters

Even though anxiety stems from many factors that have nothing to do with money, financial stress is real and can be just as tormenting as other types of stress that exists. Debt, in particular, is a major reason why people commonly feel anxiety, and this can be a stressful problem for many reasons. We all want to appear like we can purchase the little pleasantries in life, like a night out with friends or the ability to go on a date with our loved one every once in a while. To eliminate financial anxiety from your life, it's important that you can look at your finances from a straightforward lens. Be honest with yourself. What are you spending money on that is excessive or downright silly? Some great ways to eliminate excessive payments include getting rid of your cable and opting to use streaming services like Netflix instead, canceling online subscriptions that you never use, and even calling your insurance companies and figuring out if they can offer you lower rates.

Go to Bed Early, and Wake Up Early

When you have trouble sleeping, it can often seem like your next day has been ruined. You wake up feeling tired, and you spend the rest of the day feeling irritable because you did not get enough sleep the night before. Yes, anxiety can come from not getting enough sleep at night, but a lack of sleep could be affecting your ability to deal with anxiety more than you think. If you have trouble sleeping, the best advice is to try and alter your sleeping habits before turning to addictive medicines or therapy. You can start by committing to waking up just fifteen minutes earlier than you normally do each day. At night, go to bed fifteen minutes earlier than usual. While you will probably be tired at first, this will allow you to work towards more positive sleeping habits on a regular basis. You may find that over time, you will feel more tired in the evening, making it easier to fall asleep (as long as you do not take a nap during the day!)

Chapter 10
Common Mistakes to Avoid When Navigating Your Stress

You can look at this chapter as an extension of the previous chapter in the sense that both chapters can offer you valuable advice on how to permanently eliminate excessive stress from your life. Specifically, this chapter is going to discuss common mistakes that people will often make when they are looking to alleviate anxiety. The hope is that after reading this chapter, you will be much less likely to make these mistakes yourself.

Mistake to Avoid 1: Hesitation

A large portion of anxiety involves being fearful of uncertain things in life. Perhaps the most critical mistake the people with excessive anxiety make is that they will only act when they feel as if they are one-hundred percent and completely ready to do so. While being prepared is a positive thing in life, being fearful of potentially negative outcomes to the point of hesitation is not a positive in any sense of the word. To get over this type of behavior, take some time to think about the worst possible outcome first, then the best possible outcome, and then finally the most realistic outcome. The goal when you think in this manner is to reveal to yourself that both negative, as well as positive outcomes, are entirely possible.

Mistake to Avoid 2: Dodging Criticism

People who suffer from anxiety are also typically hypercritical of themselves. For this reason, anxiety-ridden people can often seek to avoid criticism at all costs. Another reason why anxious people avoid criticism is that after they have been criticized, they will spend the rest of their day going over the criticisms that they have received. While this can be a difficult tendency to overcome, a great way to do so is by faking your positive acknowledgment of criticism when you are faced with it. For example, when you are being presented with criticism, either through a job or through some other type of situation, try to meet it with a smile and approachable body posture. If you have ever heard the phrase, "fake it 'til you make it", this is a similar approach. Even if you are inwardly cringing while the criticism is occurring, an outward appearance of gratitude for the criticism can make the entire exchange more pleasant and positive.

Mistake to Avoid 3: Never Slowing Down

This mistake is something that almost everyone who lives in modern American society is guilty of committing. From the time that we wake up until the time that we go to sleep, we are constantly being bombarded by advertisements and countless other technological stimuli that encourage us to not only be in a constant state of never feeling like we're doing enough. Fulfillment in life does not need to come from our things, yet we often look to the constant acquisition of physical possessions as a way to make our lives more fulfilling. If you find that you are constantly working towards a goal of needing more money to buy more things, re-evaluating how happy these things actually make you happy is a great way to alleviate unwanted anxiety.

Mistake to Avoid 4: Looking to Others for Validation

In addition to being constantly on the move, another potential problem that can sometimes lead to large amounts of anxiety have to do with social media applications that are extremely popular in today's society. Everyone wants to show everyone else their latest travel destination, their latest engagement ring, and their newest baby that they have recently had. When you start comparing yourself to these types of people by asking yourself questions like, "when's the last time I went on a vacation?" or begin to think thoughts along the lines of, "Jeez, I wonder when my boyfriend is going to propose to me" and "I really need to think about buying a house soon", you can truly put yourself in a stressful situation within seconds.

A great way to combat the anxiety that comes with FOMO (fear of missing out) is to take at least one day to unplug from your social media applications. One day may not seem like much, but you can start with one day and then work towards adding more days without social media into your weekly schedule. If you commit to this type of habit, you are likely going to find that you notice a lot more about the world that you are living in when you are not constantly on your phone checking up on your friends and family. Additionally, you should also take note of how your anxiety decreases when you choose to distance yourself from your social media applications.

Again, this chapter, as well as the previous chapter, was meant to provide you with sound advice on how to alleviate your anxiety over the long-term. You do not have to be in competition with friends and even family members in your life who seem to "have it all together"; yet, it's very easy to get caught up in comparing yourself to others. By simply stepping back, becoming more confident and opening yourself up to your potential as a person, your anxiety is sure to lessen at least some degree.

Conclusion

Congratulations on making it to the end of this book, *Anxiety: A Beginner's Guide to Deal with It*. Hopefully, this book has been able to provide you with valuable information regarding everything that comes with having large amounts of anxiety. Remember, anxiety can be both an internal struggle that can lead to external consequences when it's not dealt with in a healthy manner. This is why it's important to take the advice that was presented in this book, especially if you feel large levels of anxiety on a regular basis. Additionally, it's important that you seek out professional help if you feel like you are largely unable to deal with your anxiety in a healthy manner. Sometimes, talking to someone on a weekly basis can make the difference between feeling levelheaded and feeling confused, nervous, and scared.

This book is a practical guide on how you can best deal with anxiety. We've gone over what anxiety is, the main types of anxiety that people suffer from, and techniques that you can use to rid yourself of anxiety over the long term. Using these techniques by themselves is often not enough for someone to rid themselves of anxiety over the long-term. A positive attitude, patience, and a firm dedication to getting rid of your anxiety are also required. While this book presented the various types of anxiety in a straightforward and easy-to-interpret fashion, it's also important to note that you could potentially experience symptoms from multiple types of anxiety. Your anxiety is unique, and thus you should try to figure out its nuances as best as possible. This way, you can work to abolish effectively.

Lastly, thank you for purchasing this book! A review on Amazon is always appreciated!

www.ingramcontent.com/pod-product-compliance
Lightning Source LLC
Chambersburg PA
CBHW050018230526
45470CB00003B/1024